HOW TO TRAIN A DOG

The Ultimate Guide to Positive Reinforcement Training for a Well-Behaved Pup.

GIFT BRIGHT

TABLE OF CONTENTS

CHAPTETR 1

Introduction to Dog Training

1.1 Understanding the Importance of Dog Training

Dog training is the process of teaching dogs specific behaviors and commands. It is an essential aspect of responsible pet ownership and plays a crucial role in maintaining a harmonious relationship between dogs and their owners. Training not only helps in preventing unwanted behaviors but also promotes positive interactions, enhances communication, and strengthens the bond between dogs and their owners.

1.2 Benefits of Training Your Dog

There are numerous benefits to training your dog. Here are some key advantages:

1.2.1 Improved Behavior: Training helps in teaching dogs appropriate behaviors and manners, such as walking on a leash, sitting, staying, and coming when called. This leads to a well-behaved dog that is easier to manage and live with.

1.2.2 Enhanced Safety: Training your dog to respond to commands like "stay" or "come" can be crucial in potentially dangerous situations. It ensures their safety and prevents them from running into traffic or getting into other hazardous situations.

1.2.3 Socialization: Training allows dogs to interact with other dogs and people in a controlled environment, promoting positive socialization. This helps reduce fear, anxiety, and aggression, making them more comfortable and well-adjusted in various situations.

1.2.4 Mental Stimulation: Dogs are intelligent animals that require mental stimulation to prevent boredom and destructive behaviors. Training provides mental exercise, challenges their problem-solving abilities, and keeps them mentally engaged.

1.2.5 Strengthened Bond: Training sessions involve positive reinforcement and bonding time with your dog. This strengthens the bond between you and your pet, creating a trusting and loving relationship.

1.2.6 Stress Reduction: Dogs that receive proper training are generally less stressed and anxious. They understand what is expected of them and feel more secure in their environment, leading to a happier and more relaxed dog.

1.2.7 Good Citizenship: Well-trained dogs are more likely to be accepted in public places, such as parks, cafes, and stores. They are less likely to cause disturbances or engage in disruptive behaviors, making them good canine citizens.

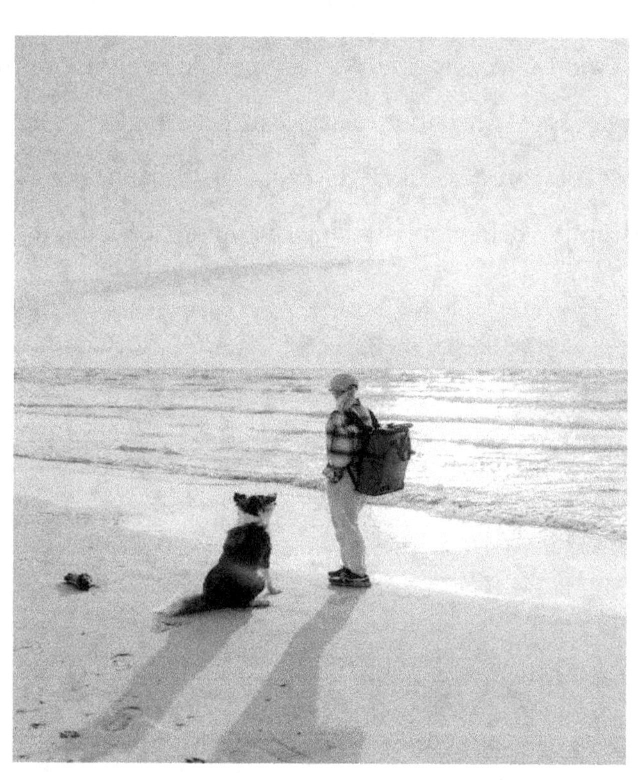

CHAPTER 2

Preparing for Dog Training

2.1 Setting Realistic Expectations

Before starting dog training, it is important to set realistic expectations. Understand that every dog is unique and learns at their own pace. Some dogs may pick up commands quickly, while others may require more time and patience. It is fundamental to show restraint, predictable, and understanding all through the preparation interaction. Setting realistic goals and understanding that progress may be gradual will help you stay motivated and focused.

2.2 Gathering Necessary Training Supplies

To effectively train your dog, you will need certain training supplies. Here are some essential items:

2.2.1 Treats: High-value treats are a great motivator for dogs during training sessions. Choose small, soft, and easily chewable treats that your dog finds irresistible.

2.2.2 Clicker: A clicker is a small handheld device that makes a distinct clicking sound. It is used as a marker to indicate when your dog has performed the desired behavior correctly. Clickers are commonly used in positive reinforcement training.

2.2.3 Leash and Collar/Harness: A leash and collar or harness are necessary for teaching your dog leash manners and basic commands. Choose a leash and collar/harness that is appropriate for your dog's size and breed.

2.2.4 Training Pads or Litter Box: If you are training your dog to eliminate indoors, training pads or a litter box specifically designed for dogs can be useful.

2.2.5 Toys: Interactive toys can be used as rewards during training sessions or to keep your dog mentally stimulated outside of training.

2.2.6 Treat Pouch or Training Bag: A treat pouch or training bag allows you to conveniently carry treats during training sessions, keeping them easily accessible.

2.3 Creating a Positive Training Environment

Creating a positive training environment is crucial for successful dog training. Here are some tips:

2.3.1 Choose a Quiet and Distraction-Free Area: Find a quiet area in your home or yard where you can conduct training sessions without distractions. This will help your dog focus better and improve their learning experience.

2.3.2 Use Positive Reinforcement: Positive reinforcement involves rewarding your dog for performing the desired behavior. This can be done through treats, praise, petting, or play. Avoid using punishment or harsh methods, as they can damage the trust and bond between you and your dog.

2.3.3 Set Aside Regular Training Time: Consistency is key when it comes to training. Set aside regular, dedicated training time to work with your dog. Short, frequent sessions are generally more effective than long, infrequent ones.

2.3.4 Be Patient and Consistent: Dogs learn through repetition and consistency. Be patient with your dog and consistently reinforce the desired behaviors. Avoid getting frustrated or giving up if progress seems slow. Remember, training takes time and effort.

2.3.5 Keep Training Sessions Short and Fun: Dogs have short attention spans, so keep training sessions short, usually around 5-10 minutes, and end them on a positive note. Make training fun and engaging for your dog to keep them motivated and eager to learn.

By setting realistic expectations, gathering necessary training supplies, and creating a positive training environment, you will be well-prepared to begin your dog training journey. Remember to be patient, consistent, and positive throughout the process, and enjoy the bonding experience with your furry friend.

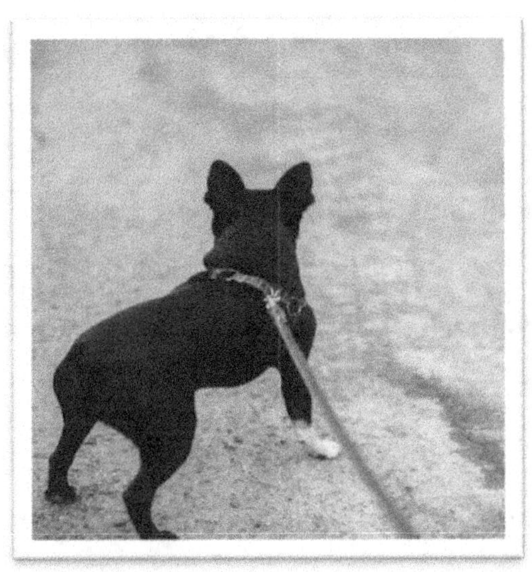

Leash and Collar/Harness

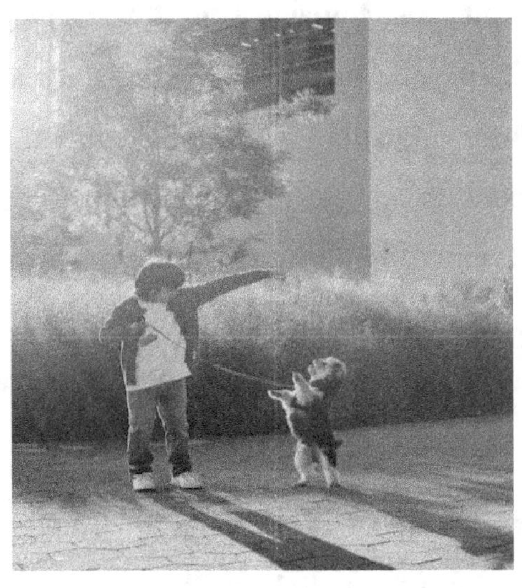

CHAPTER 3

Basic Dog Training Techniques

3.1 Establishing Leadership and Building Trust: In order to effectively train your dog, it's important to establish yourself as the leader. This can be done through consistent rules and boundaries, as well as positive reinforcement and building trust with your dog.

3.2 Teaching Basic Commands (Sit, Stay, Lie Down): Start by teaching your dog the basic commands such as sit, stay, and lie down. Use treats and positive reinforcement to encourage your dog to perform these commands. In your training, be persistent and patient. **3.3 Using Positive Reinforcement:** Positive reinforcement involves rewarding your dog for good behavior. Treats, compliments, or playing can do this. By rewarding your dog when they exhibit desired behavior, you are reinforcing that behavior and encouraging them to repeat it.

3.4 Implementing Clicker Training: Clicker training is a technique that uses a clicker to mark desired behavior, followed by a reward. The clicker serves as a signal to the dog that they have done something correctly. This method can be effective in teaching new behaviors or reinforcing existing ones.

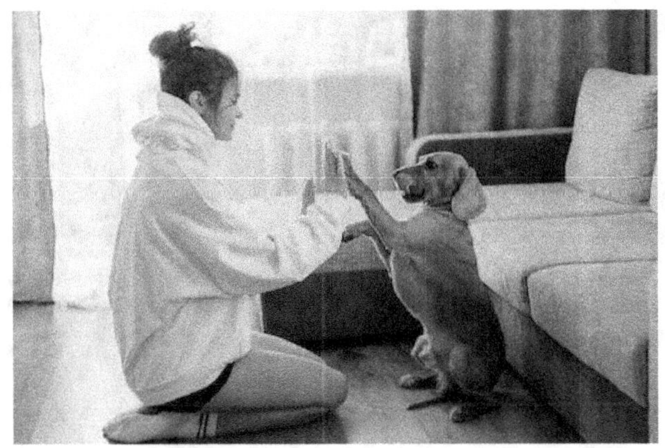

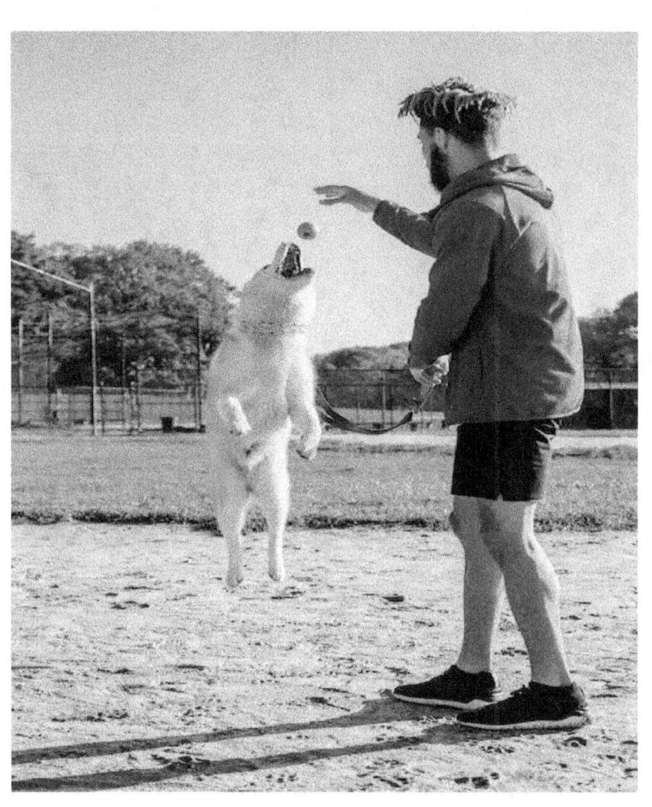

CHAPTER 4

Socializing Your Dog

4.1 The Importance of Socialization: Socialization is crucial for dogs to develop good behavior and proper social skills. It helps them feel comfortable in various environments and interact positively with other dogs and people.

4.2 Introducing Your Dog to New Environments: Gradually expose your dog to different environments, such as parks, streets, and public places. Start with quieter areas and gradually increase the level of distraction. They will get more acclimated to unfamiliar sights, sounds, and scents as a result.

4.3 Encouraging Positive Interactions with Other Dogs and People: Allow your dog to interact with other dogs and people in a controlled and positive manner. Start with calm and friendly dogs, and gradually introduce them to different sizes, breeds, and temperaments. Encourage positive interactions and reward good behavior.

Remember to always prioritize your dog's safety and comfort during socialization. Take it slow and provide positive reinforcement to help your dog feel confident and well-adjusted in various social situations.

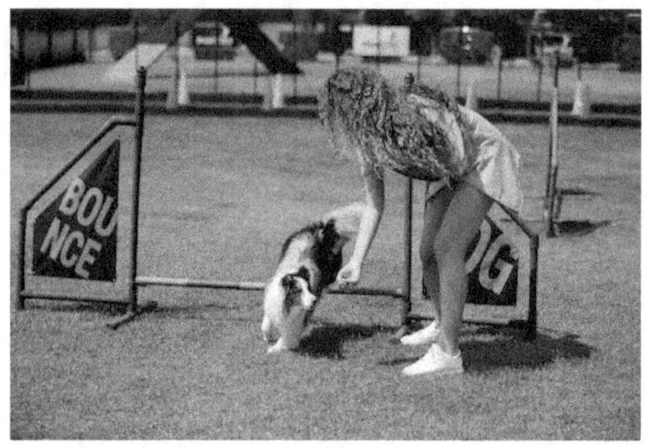

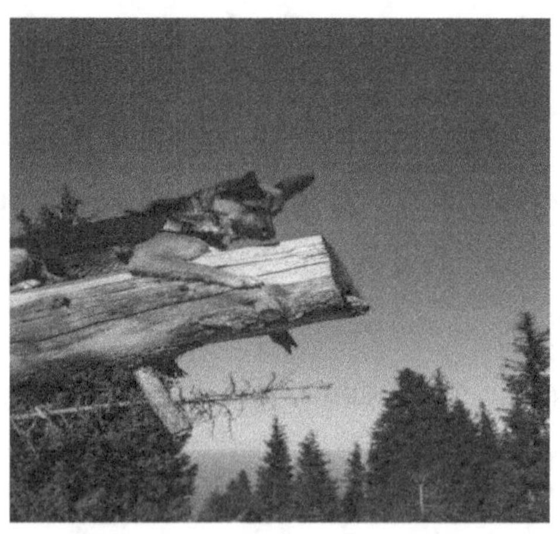

CHAPTER 5

Addressing Common Behavior Issues

5.1 Dealing with Barking Problems: Identify the cause of excessive barking, such as boredom, fear, or alerting to something. Use positive reinforcement to reward quiet behavior and provide mental and physical stimulation to prevent boredom.

5.2 Handling Separation Anxiety: Gradually desensitize your dog to being alone by leaving them alone for short periods and gradually increasing the duration. Provide them with comforting items, such as a favorite toy or blanket, and create a calm and safe environment.

5.3 Managing Leash Pulling and Walking Etiquette: Teach your dog loose leash walking by rewarding them for walking calmly beside you. Use positive reinforcement and redirect their attention when they start pulling. Consistency and patience are key in teaching proper leash manners.

5.4 Correcting Jumping and Nipping Behaviors: Teach your dog alternative behaviors, such as sitting or offering a toy, to redirect their jumping or nipping behavior. Ignore the unwanted behavior and reward them for calm and appropriate behavior. Consistency and positive reinforcement are important in addressing these issues.

Always keep in mind that treating behavior problems needs tolerance, perseverance, and encouragement. It's also important to understand that each dog is unique, so tailor your training approach to suit your dog's individual needs.

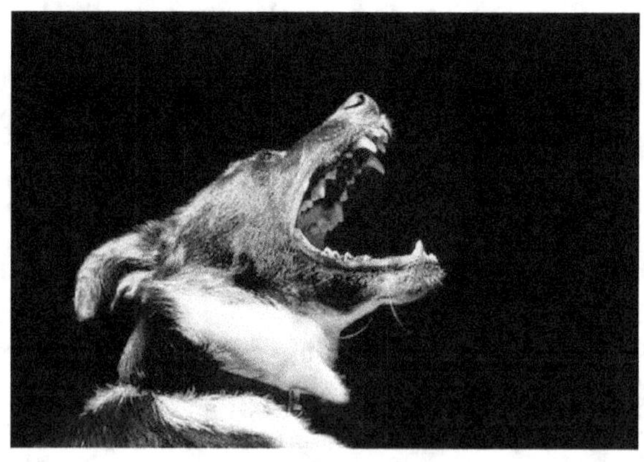

CHAPTER 6

Advanced Training Techniques

6.1 Teaching Advanced Commands (Fetch, Roll Over, etc.): Once your dog has mastered the basic commands, you can move on to teaching them more advanced commands like fetch, roll over, or play dead. Break down these commands into smaller steps and use positive reinforcement to encourage your dog's progress.

6.2 Training for Specific Tasks (Agility, Search and Rescue, etc.): If you have specific tasks in mind for your dog, such as agility training or search and rescue work, seek professional guidance or join specialized training classes. These activities require specialized training techniques and guidance to ensure both you and your dog's safety.

6.3 Training for Canine Sports and Competitions: If you're interested in participating in canine sports or competitions, research the specific requirements and training techniques for those activities. Seek guidance from experienced trainers and consider joining training clubs or organizations that focus on the specific sport or competition you're interested in.

Remember to always prioritize your dog's well-being and enjoyment during advanced training. Use positive reinforcement, break down tasks into manageable steps, and seek professional guidance when needed. Enjoy the journey of advanced training with your dog.

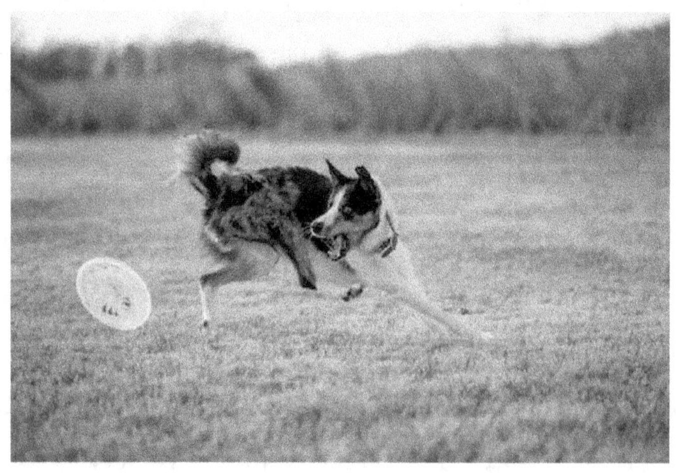

CHAPTER 7

Maintaining Training Consistency

7.1 Implementing Regular Training Sessions: Set aside dedicated time each day for training sessions with your dog. Try to build a schedule that works for both you and your dog since consistency is important. Keep training sessions short and enjoyable to maintain your dog's focus and motivation.

7.2 Reinforcing Training Throughout Daily Life: Training shouldn't be limited to formal sessions. Take advantage of everyday situations to reinforce the training your dog has learned. For example, ask your dog to sit before mealtime or before going for a walk. This helps reinforce their training and keeps their skills sharp.

7.3 Troubleshooting Training Challenges: It's common to face challenges during training. If you encounter difficulties, take a step back and evaluate the situation. Assess if there are any underlying issues or if adjustments need to be made to your training methods. Seek guidance from a professional trainer if needed, as they can provide valuable insights and solutions.

Remember, consistency is key in maintaining training progress. Regular training sessions, reinforcement throughout daily life, and addressing challenges as they arise will help you and your dog achieve long-term success in training. Keep up the good work.

CHAPTER 8

Continuing Education for You and Your Dog

8.1 Exploring Further Training Resources: There are numerous books, online courses, videos, and articles available that can provide further training resources for you and your dog. Explore different training methods, techniques, and theories to expand your knowledge and find what works best for you and your dog.

8.2 Participating in Dog Training Classes or Workshops: Consider enrolling in dog training classes or workshops to further enhance your training skills and provide your dog with socialization opportunities. These classes are often led by experienced trainers who can provide guidance, feedback, and support as you continue your training journey.

8.3 Seeking Professional Training Assistance if Needed: If you encounter specific challenges or feel overwhelmed, don't hesitate to seek professional training assistance. A professional dog trainer can provide personalized guidance, tailored training plans, and address any specific behavior issues you may be facing.

Continuing education is important for both you and your dog to ensure ongoing growth and development. Explore different resources, participate in training classes or workshops, and seek professional assistance when needed. Enjoy the journey of learning and training with your dog.

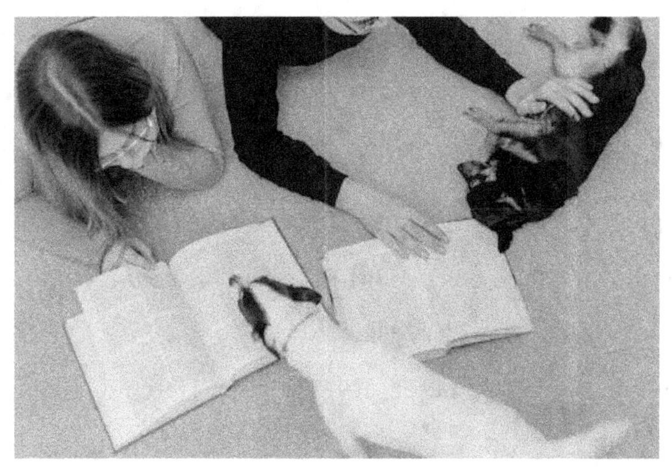

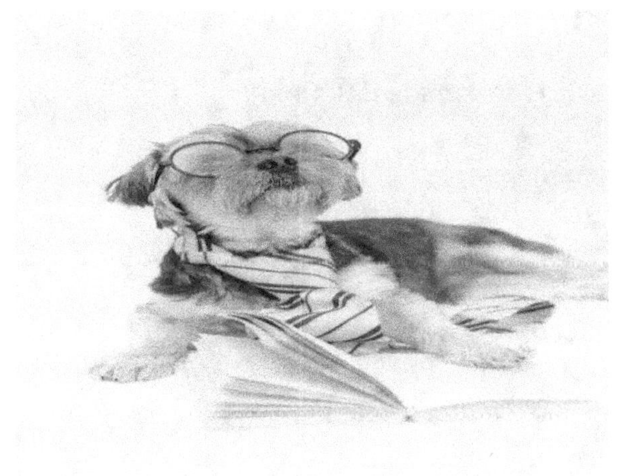

CHAPTER 9

Dog Meal Plan

Feeding your dog a well-balanced and nutritious diet is essential for their overall health and well-being. Creating a meal plan for your furry friend can be a great way to ensure they receive all the necessary nutrients. Here are some dog meal plan recipes, along with their ingredients and preparation methods

Day 1:

Breakfast: Homemade dog food

Ingredients:

- 1 cup cooked brown rice

- 1/2 cup cooked ground turkey

- 1/2 cup cooked green beans

- 1/4 cup chopped carrots

- 1 tablespoon olive oil

Prep method:

1. Cook the earthy colored rice as per bundle guidelines.

2. Cook the ground turkey in a pan until it is no longer pink.

3. In a separate pan, cook the green beans and carrots until they are tender.

4. Combine all ingredients in a mixing bowl and mix well.

5. Serve to your dog.

Lunch: Chicken and Rice

Ingredients:

- 1/2 cup cooked brown rice

- 1/2 cup cooked shredded chicken

- 1/4 cup chopped broccoli

- 1 tablespoon olive oil

Prep method:

1. Cook the brown rice following package instructions.

2. Cook the chicken in a pan until it is no longer pink.

3. In a separate pan, cook the broccoli until it is tender.

4. Combine all ingredients in a mixing bowl and mix well.

5. Serve to your dog.

Dinner: Beef and Sweet Potato Stew

Ingredients:

- 1/2 pound ground beef

- 1 sweet potato, peeled and chopped

- 1/2 cup chopped carrots

- 1/2 cup chopped green beans

- 1 tablespoon olive oil

Prep method:

1. Cook the ground beef in a pan until it is no longer pink.

2. In a separate pan, cook the sweet potato, carrots, and green beans until they are tender.

3. Combine all ingredients in a slow cooker and cook on low for 6 hours.

4. Serve to your dog.

Day 2:

Breakfast: Yogurt and Blueberries

Ingredients:

- 1/2 cup plain Greek yogurt

- 1/4 cup blueberries

Prep method:

1. Mix the yogurt and blueberries together in a bowl.

2. Serve to your dog.

Lunch: Tuna and Rice

Ingredients:

- 1/2 cup cooked brown rice

- 1 can of tuna, drained

- 1/4 cup chopped carrots

- 1 tablespoon olive oil

Prep method:

1. Prepare the brown rice as directed on the box.

2. In a mixing bowl, combine the cooked rice, tuna, and chopped carrots.

3. Mix well.

4. Serve to your dog.

Dinner: Turkey and Sweet Potato Mash

Ingredients:

- 1/2 pound ground turkey

- 1 sweet potato, peeled and chopped

- 1/4 cup chopped green beans

- 1 tablespoon olive oil

Prep method:

1. Cook the ground turkey in a pan until it is no longer pink.

2. In a separate pan, cook the sweet potato and green beans until they are tender.

3. Combine all ingredients in a mixing bowl and mash together.

4. Serve to your dog.

Day 3:

Breakfast: Banana and Peanut Butter Oatmeal

Ingredients:

- 1/2 cup cooked oatmeal

- 1/2 banana, sliced

- 1 tablespoon peanut butter

Prep method:

1. Cook the oatmeal according to package instructions.

2. Mix in the sliced banana and peanut butter.

3. Serve to your dog.

Lunch: Chicken and Vegetable Stir Fry

Ingredients:

- 1/2 cup cooked brown rice

- 1/2 cup cooked shredded chicken

- 1/4 cup chopped broccoli

- 1/4 cup chopped carrots

- 1 tablespoon olive oil

Prep method:

1. Cook the brown rice according to package instructions.

2. In a pan, heat the olive oil and add the chicken and vegetables.

3. Cook until the vegetables are tender.

4. Serve over the cooked brown rice.

Dinner: Beef and Vegetable Soup

Ingredients:

- 1/2 pound ground beef

- 1/2 cup chopped carrots

- 1/2 cup chopped green beans

- 1/2 cup chopped potatoes

- 1 tablespoon olive oil

- 4 cups low-sodium beef broth

Prep method:

1. Cook the ground beef in a pan until it is no longer pink.

2. In a separate pot, heat the olive oil and add the chopped vegetables.

3. Cook until the vegetables are tender.

4. Add the cooked ground beef and beef broth to the pot.

5. Bring to a boil, then reduce heat and simmer for 30 minutes.

6. Serve to your dog.

Day 4:

Breakfast: Scrambled Eggs and Cheese

Ingredients:

- 2 eggs

- 1/4 cup shredded cheese

Prep method:

1. In a mixing dish, crack the eggs and stir them in.

2. Heat a pan over medium heat and add the egg mixture.

3. Cook until the eggs are scrambled and no longer runny.

4. Sprinkle shredded cheese on top and cook until melted.

5. Serve to your dog.

Lunch: Turkey and Vegetable Casserole

Ingredients:

- 1/2 pound ground turkey

- 1/2 cup chopped broccoli

- 1/2 cup chopped carrots

- 1/2 cup chopped sweet potatoes

- 1 tablespoon olive oil

Prep method:

1. Cook the ground turkey in a pan until it is no longer pink.

2. In a separate pan, cook the vegetables until they are tender.

3. Combine the cooked turkey and vegetables in a casserole dish.

4. 20 minutes of baking at 350 degrees Fahrenheit.

5. Serve to your dog.

Dinner: Salmon and Sweet Potato Cakes

Ingredients:

- 1 can of salmon, drained and flaked

- 1 sweet potato, peeled and grated

- 1/4 cup chopped green beans

- 1 tablespoon olive oil

Prep method:

1. In a mixing bowl, combine the salmon, grated sweet potato, and chopped green beans.

2. Mix well.

3. Form the mixture into patties.

4. Heat the olive oil in a pan over medium heat.

5. Cook the patties for 3-4 minutes on each side, until golden brown.

6. Serve to your dog.

Day 5:

Breakfast: Blueberry and Banana Smoothie

Ingredients:

- 1/2 cup plain Greek yogurt

- 1/2 banana

- 1/4 cup blueberries

- 1/4 cup water

Prep method:

1. Utilizing a blender, combine all ingredients and process until smooth.

2. Serve to your dog.

Lunch: Beef and Vegetable Stew

Ingredients:

- 1/2 pound stew beef

- 1/2 cup chopped carrots

- 1/2 cup chopped green beans

- 1/2 cup chopped potatoes

- 1 tablespoon olive oil

- 4 cups low-sodium beef broth

Prep method:

1. Cook the stew beef in a pan until it is browned on all sides.

2. In a separate pot, heat the olive oil and add the chopped vegetables.

3. Cook until the vegetables are tender.

4. Add the cooked beef and beef broth to the pot.

5. Bring to a boil, then reduce heat and simmer for 30 minutes.

6. Serve to your dog.

Dinner: Chicken and Quinoa

Ingredients:

- 1/2 cup cooked quinoa

- 1/2 cup cooked shredded chicken

- 1/4 cup chopped sweet potatoes

- 1 tablespoon olive oil

Prep method:

1. To prepare the quinoa, follow the directions on the box.

2. Cook the shredded chicken in a pan until it is no longer pink.

3. In a separate pan, cook the sweet potatoes until they are tender.

4. Combine all ingredients in a mixing bowl and mix well.

5. Serve to your dog.

Day 6:

Breakfast: Peanut Butter and Banana Oatmeal

Ingredients:

- 1/2 cup cooked oatmeal

- 1/2 banana, sliced

- 1 tablespoon peanut butter

Prep method:

1. Cook the oatmeal according to package instructions.

2. Mix in the sliced banana and peanut butter.

3. Serve to your dog.

Lunch: Tuna and Vegetable Salad

Ingredients:

- 1 can of tuna, drained

- 1/4 cup chopped carrots

- 1/4 cup chopped green beans

- 1/4 cup chopped broccoli

- 1 tablespoon olive oil

Prep method:

1. In a mixing bowl, combine the drained tuna and chopped vegetables.

2. Mix well.

3. Drizzle with olive oil and mix again.

4. Serve to your dog.

Dinner: Beef and Sweet Potato Hash

Ingredients:

- 1/2 pound ground beef

- 1 sweet potato, peeled and chopped

- 1/4 cup chopped green beans

- 1 tablespoon olive oil

Prep method:

1. Cook the ground beef in a pan until it is no longer pink.

2. In a separate pan, cook the sweet potato and green beans until they are tender.

3. Combine all ingredients in a mixing bowl and mix well.

4. Serve to your dog.

Day 7:

Breakfast: Cottage Cheese and Blueberries

Ingredients:

- 1/2 cup cottage cheese

- 1/4 cup blueberries

Prep method:

1. Mix the cottage cheese and blueberries together in a bowl.

2. Serve to your dog.

Lunch: Chicken and Rice Soup

Ingredients:

- 1/2 cup cooked brown rice

- 1/2 cup cooked shredded chicken

- 1/4 cup chopped carrots

- 1/4 cup chopped celery

- 4 cups low-sodium chicken broth

Prep method:

1. According to the directions on the package, prepare the brown rice.

2. In a pot, heat the chicken broth and add the shredded chicken, chopped carrots, and chopped celery.

3. Cook until the vegetables are tender.

4. Add the cooked brown rice to the pot and stir.

5. Serve to your dog.

Dinner: Turkey and Vegetable Skewers

Ingredients:

- 1/2 pound ground turkey

- 1/4 cup chopped zucchini

- 1/4 cup chopped bell pepper

- 1/4 cup chopped onion

- 1 tablespoon olive oil

Prep method:

1. Set the oven's temperature to 350 degrees Fahrenheit.

2. In a mixing bowl, combine the ground turkey and chopped vegetables.

3. Mix well.

4. Form the mixture into small balls and place on skewers.

5. Brush with olive oil.

6. Bake in the oven for 20-25 minutes, or until cooked through.

7. Serve to your dog.

Conclusion

9.1 Recap of Key Training Principles: Throughout this guide, we have discussed various training techniques, including establishing leadership, teaching basic commands, socializing your dog, addressing behavior issues, advanced training techniques, maintaining training consistency, and continuing education. Key principles include consistency, patience, positive reinforcement, and seeking professional guidance when needed.

9.2 Celebrating Your Dog's Progress: Training your dog is a journey that requires time, effort, and dedication. It's important to celebrate your dog's progress along the way. Acknowledge and reward their achievements, no matter how small. Remember that every dog learns at their own pace, so be patient and understanding.

By following these training techniques and principles, you can strengthen the bond with your dog, improve their behavior, and create a harmonious and fulfilling relationship. Enjoy the process of training and growing together with your dog,